Lose Weight With

Hypnotherapy

or NOT!!

by Walker O'Duggan, MA, CACHt

CONTENTS

Forward

So you want to lose weight. No big surprise there. Well, seems like about 90% of all Americans want to lose some weight whether it be 5 pounds or 50 pounds. I wanted to lose 30 pounds about a year ago and I was able to lose 28 of the 30 pounds and I'm happy with where I'm at now. I didn't use a diet. I didn't starve myself and I didn't listen to other people with their opinions of how they lost weight. Because the people that I had to listen to were all still overweight. Sure they had lost weight on a diet but they've gained all that weight back and in most cases had gained back even more than they lost originally. So I did it the old-fashioned way. Cold Turkey and hypnosis. I know that most people that read this are searching for a silver bullet or a quick fix. But it took you years to gain the weight so it's going to take some time to lose it. I've included a typical diet for those of you who read this book but are afraid, or will not go to a hypnotherapist. I do recommend the hypnotherapist in order to lose weight properly however I understand that not everyone agrees with our feels the same way that I do about hypnotherapy. So go ahead and read this book and determine which part of it you'll use and which part you won't use. Their is something in here for everyone who is trying to lose weight.

I remember back in 1963 when I joined the Marine Corps. I believe, I weighed 121 pounds. After boot camp I was down to 114 pounds. Most people in Marine Corps boot camp gain weight because of all of the extra food. I actually lost weight because I wasn't used to the exercise that was required. I guess what happened was the old adage "calories in calories out." I may have been taking in 3000 cal a day but I was burning 5000. Then in 1965,when I went to Vietnam. I weighed about 130 pounds when I came home I weighing 110 pounds and again calories in calories out. I know that C rations didn't have a really good flavor, but they were the only thing that was semi editable. I tried eating some of the water buffalo skin and the fried snails and even once ate dog meat and none of that was to my liking. So, as a pampered American I was unable to keep Vietnamese cuisine down. It appeared to me that the only thing I was going to be able to keep down was C rations. More often than not I wasn't even able to keep the C rations down, but this story isn't about me and my experiences in Vietnam or my experiences trying to gain weight. This book is about you and how hypnotherapy can help you lose the weight that you're trying to lose. I guess basically what I'm trying to tell you is "calories in calories out." If you can change the way that you think, you can change your destiny.

When I came home from the war. I was so thin that my friends who had come home months or years before me or who had never gone over there were all of normal weight to height, but to me they looked like overly robust American men. I on the other hand was still extremely slim. I got a job in law enforcement.

So naturally I started to lift weights with my friends on my shift. One especially who was a professional weightlifter and a Mr. Olympia contestant, Doug Betts suggested that I try a high-protein milkshake called MLO. This did of course help me gain weight and I probably got up to about 140 pounds. I was working as a deputy sheriff, so I was setting in my car more than I was running after the criminals. I would occasionally go out and run in order to stay in shape, however between the milkshakes and the extra food that I was eating trying to gain weight. I was really not gaining much. Now that I'm over 60 years old. It seems that all that weight. I tried to gain when I was younger has come on with a vengeance. Now I work at keeping the weight off. So let's do this book on how to lose weight.

Diet and Health

Preliminary Bout

Rule to Finding the Ideal Adult Net Weight

Multiply number of inches over 5 ft. in height by 6.0; add 110. For example: Height 5 ft. 7 in. without shoes.

7 x 6.0 = 42 + 110 ------- Ideal weight 152 lbs.

If under 5 ft. multiply number of inches under 5 ft. by 6 and subtract from 110.

Is your weight where it should be or are you too heavy.

Now fat individuals have always been considered a joke, but you are a joke no longer. Instead of being looked upon with friendly tolerance and amusement, you are now viewed with distrust, suspicion, and even aversion! How dare you hoard fat. Why you don't dare to any longer. You never wanted to be fat anyway, but you did not know how to reduce, and it is proverbial how little you eat. Why, there is the beautiful young girl in the office, who is extremely thin, and she eats twice as much as you do, and does not gain an ounce. You know positively that eating has nothing to do with it, the many times that you dieted, didn't eat a thing but what the doctor ordered, besides your regular meals, and you actually gained.

You are in despair about being anything but fat, and--! how you hate it. But cheer up. I will save you, even as I have saved myself and many, many others, so will I save you. You're wanting to lose weight has to be a desire so strong that you're willing to do anything to achieve your goal. As always you can buy my books for more info on different subjects.   I suggest hypnotherapy. Find yourself a good hypnotist set an appointment and do exactly what they tell you to do and I guarantee you if you have the desire to lose weight and you see hypnotherapist you will lose weight.

Jolly Mrs. Cheesecake has the floor and wants some questions answered. You know Mrs. Cheesecake; her husband recently bought her a pair of freight scales.

You may ask this question or you may have asked this question many times "Why is it, , that thin people can eat so much more than fat people and still not gain?"

"First: Thin people are usually more active than fat people and use up their calories. Remember calories in calories out.

"Second: Thin people have been proved to radiate fifty per cent more heat per pound than fat people; in other words, fat people are regular fire-less cookers! They hold the heat in, it cannot get out through the packing.

"And , then there are baby fire-less cookers and children fire-less cookers. The same dietetic rules apply to them as to the adult."

"We have heard people say that fat people are fat because, they eat too much, when the truth is that we eat so little?"

"Yes, you eat too much, *no matter how little it is*, even if it be only one bird-seed daily, *if you store it away as fat*.

"But, you say, is it not true that some individuals inherit the tendency to be fat, and can not help it, no matter what they do?"

"Answer to first part--Yes.

"Answer to second part--No! It is not true that they cannot help it; they have to work a little harder, that is all. It is true that being fat is a disease with some, due to imperfect working of the internal secreter glands, such as the thyroid, generative glands, etc.; but that is not true fat such as you have. Yours, and that of the other people who are interested, is due to overeating and under exercising.

"Those diseased individuals should be under the care of a physician. Probably the secreter glands are somewhat inactive or sluggish in the healthy fat individual. I use the word *healthy* here in contradistinction to the other type. In reality, individuals very much overweight are not really healthy, and they should also visit their physician."

But, what's the use of dieting? I only get fatter after I stop."

Try to remember that, **weight is just a number**. If you're too fat to fit into the clothing that you like, then you need to lose weight. If you're clothes fit you properly and you feel like you look good in the mirror then you don't. So, **weight is how you feel in your mind.** I highlighted this because I want you to remember it. Remember "If you can change the way you think, you can change your destiny".

Being fat is how you feel about yourself in your mind, so being overweight is 90% in your mind and 10% in your body so through hypnotherapy, we can change how you look in your minds eye in that mirror in your mind. Through hypnotherapy. If you change the way you think you can change your destiny. I know that I have said this several times, but I want you to believe it as much as I do. I believe with all my heart that it is true.

I know everything you have to contend with--how you no sooner congratulate yourself on your will power, after you have dragged yourself by the window with an exposure of luscious fat chocolates, than another comes into view, and you have it all to go through with again, and how you finally gave in to the craving in your mind.

I hope that in the future it will be a misdemeanor, punishable by fine or imprisonment, to display candy so that the public can see it.

Many fond parents think that candy causes worms. It doesn't, of course, unless it is contaminated with worm eggs, but, personally, I wish every time I ate a chocolate I would get a worm, then I would stop eating it. The chocolates, I mean. I will tell you more about worms when I discuss meat.

I know how you go down to destruction for peanuts, with their awful fat content. It is terrible, the lure a peanut has for me. Do you suppose Mr. Darwin could explain that?

So my original question was "What's the use of dieting, If you only get fatter after you stop?

So many ask me the same question, --Will I always have to watch what I eat, for the rest of my life? And it even irritates me because I hear it so often.

The answer is,--Yes! You will always have to keep up dieting, just as you always have to keep up other things in life that make it worth living--being neat, being kind, being tender; reading, studying, loving. The only thing that will eliminate the cravings for food is hypnosis. Clinical hypnotherapy will eliminate any and all cravings. Within a few visits.

You will not feel so stressed out after you get to normal; *but you might as well recognize now, and accept it as a fact, that neither you nor anybody else will be able to eat beyond your needs without accumulating fat or disease, or both.*

WHEN YOU START TO REDUCE you will have the following to combat:

First: Your fat friends, who tells you that people do not like thin people. I almost hate them when I think how long they have kept me under that delusion. Now, of course, I know all about jealous disposition, and how they did not want me to look better than they do.

Second: Your sister, who says, "Goodness, Walker, but you look old today; you looked lots better before the diet."

Third: Your friends, who tell you that you are just right now; don't lose another pound! And other friends who tell you cheerful tales of people they have known who reduced, and who went into a decline, and finally died.

But you must not mind them. Smile, and tell them that you know all about it, and don't worry. Go serenely on your way, confident in your heart that you will look fully ten years younger when you get down to normal, no matter how you look in the interim. I don't see why women, and men, too, (secretly) worry so much about wrinkles. If the increased wrinkles on the face are accompanied by increased wrinkles in the gray matter, 'tis a consummation devoutly to be wished. I'm sure I am much more interesting with wrinkles than I was without. I am to myself, anyway.

However, you will not be any more wrinkled if you reduce gradually, as I advise, and keep up your exercises at least fifteen minutes daily.

I have a friend who recently lost 60 pounds. Prior to his weight loss. We had our photographs taken and he had to have his photograph retaken because the difference was absolutely amazing. Now when he goes into a store he looks like he needs to be carded if he tries to buy beer. Prior to the hypnotherapy session. He looked his age plus a little more, but now he looks much younger than he actually is.

Take care of your face, alternate hot and cold water, glycerin one-quarter, rose water three-quarters, cold cream packs, massage gently, a little ice--you know what to do--you need not fear. You will not only look ten years younger and live twenty years longer--I assert it boldly--but your complexion and efficiency will be one hundred per cent better. Obviously, this will also work for men but I'm not going to tell you that this is necessary because of your vanity.

If there is anything comparable to the joy of buying smaller, clothes, I have experienced it and I find it very delightful. When you find your belt coming closer to the last notch you will experience the thrill that I have experienced.

But don't be in a hurry to make your clothes smaller now. If they are loose they will show to the world that you are reducing. A fat person in a tight suit, is not something attractive, but a skinny person in baggy clothes sends a message.

I have said that calories, and calories only, causes fat. That gives you the cue to what you must do to get rid of fat. First of all, I highly recommend that if you're going to go on a diet and not use hypnotherapy, you should most certainly. First and foremost see your doctor talk to a physician and let them know what you're going to do and ascertain from them. If you're making the correct choice.

Tell your physician that you would like to start and exercise program, and when you start an exercise program start slowly especially at first, and not too frequent nor prolonged steam baths or hot tubs.

Now, if food is the only source of body substance, you see that you must study that question, and that is what I will give you--some lessons on foods and their values.

Heretofore you have known only in a dumb, despairing sort of way that all the foods you like are fattening, and all the advice you read and hear is that you must avoid them as a much as possible. And you settle down to your joyless fatness, realizing that it is beyond human strength to do that forever, and that you would rather die young and fat, anyway, than to have nothing to eat all your life but a little meat, fish, and slushy vegetables. Study on, and you will find the reason your favorite foods are fattening.

But cast off your dejection. *You don't have to avoid them*! I'm not recommending a diet only with exercise, what I am recommending is hypnotherapy eating properly and exercising.

Eat what you like and grow thin? Yes; follow me. I know it will be an exertion, but you must persist and go through with it. Nothing in life worth while is attained without some work. So begin now; it is the price of getting into that smaller dress are the smaller waistband of your trousers.

Each subject will have a review following the text so this will happen every chapter. This is your first review. So good luck.

Review

1. Give rule for normal weight.

2. How much excess food have you stored away?

3. Why more important than ever to reduce?

4. Why are fat individuals fire-less cookers?

5. Give causes of excess fat.

NOTE: The Reviews which follow the chapters are important and the questions should be answered. To get the full benefit.

This is what happens when you lose fat. Remember, **FAT IS A KILLER!**

When you lose fat...

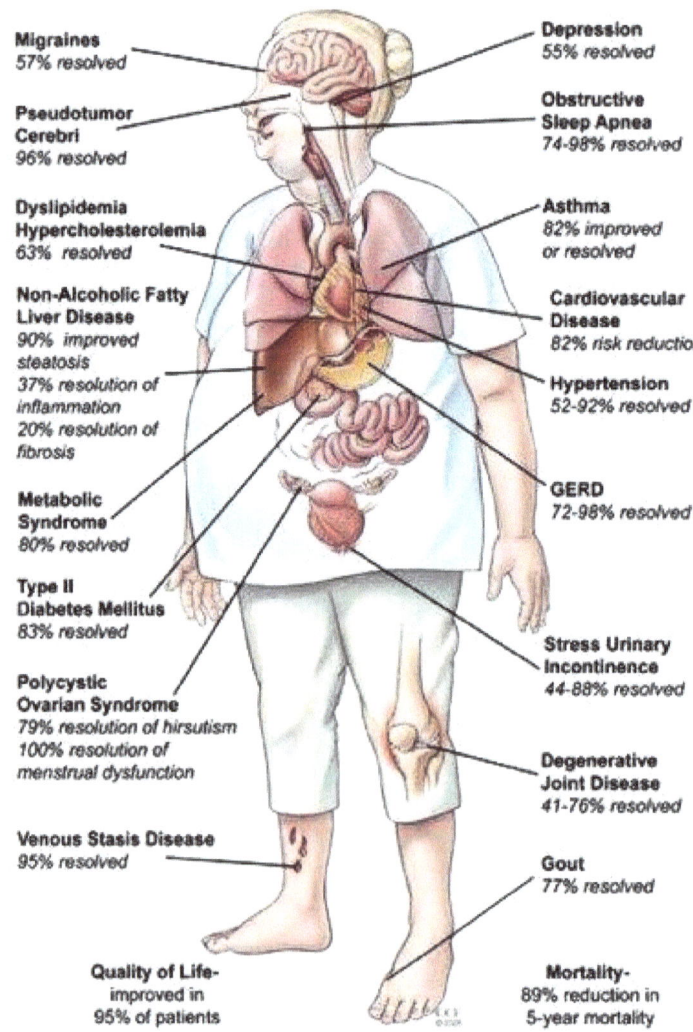

Migraines
57% resolved

Pseudotumor
Cerebri
96% resolved

Dyslipidemia
Hypercholesterolemia
63% resolved

Non-Alcoholic Fatty
Liver Disease
90% improved
steatosis
37% resolution of
inflammation
20% resolution of
fibrosis

Metabolic
Syndrome
80% resolved

Type II
Diabetes Mellitus
83% resolved

Polycystic
Ovarian Syndrome
79% resolution of hirsutism
100% resolution of
menstrual dysfunction

Venous Stasis Disease
95% resolved

Quality of Life-
improved in
95% of patients

Depression
55% resolved

Obstructive
Sleep Apnea
74-98% resolved

Asthma
82% improved
or resolved

Cardiovascular
Disease
82% risk reduction

Hypertension
52-92% resolved

GERD
72-98% resolved

Stress Urinary
Incontinence
44-88% resolved

Degenerative
Joint Disease
41-76% resolved

Gout
77% resolved

Mortality-
89% reduction in
5-year mortality

2

Key to the Calories

Definition to learn:

CALORIE; symbol C.; a heat unit and food value unit; is that amount of heat necessary to raise one pound of water 4 degrees Fahrenheit.

There is a good deal of effort expended by many semi-educated individuals to discredit the knowledge of calories, saying that it is a foolish food science, a fallacy, a fetish, and so forth.

They reason, or rather say, that because there are no calories in some of the very vital elements of foods--the vitamins and the mineral salts--therefore it is not necessary to know about them. They further argue that their grandfathers never heard of calories and they got along all right. That grandfather argument always irritates me.

Now you know that a calorie is a unit of measuring heat and food. It is not heat, not food; simply a unit of measure. And as food is of supreme importance, certainly a knowledge of how it should be measured is also of supreme importance.

You should know and also use the word calorie as frequently, or more frequently, than you use the words foot, yard, quart, gallon, and so forth, as measures of length and of liquids. Hereafter you are going to eat calories of food. Instead of saying one slice of bread, or a piece of pie, you will say 100 Calories of bread, 350 Calories of pie.

The following is the way the calorie is determined:

An apparatus known as the bomb calorimeter has two chambers, the inner, which contains the dry food to be burned, say a definite amount of sugar, and an outer, which is filled with water. The food is ignited with an electric connection and burned. This heat is transferred to the water. When one pound of water is raised 4 degrees Fahrenheit, the amount of heat used is arbitrarily chosen as the unit of heat, and is called the Calorie.

Food burned (oxidized) in the body has been proved to give off approximately the same amount of heat or energy as when burned in the calorimeter.

1 oz. Fat = 275 C. --about 255 in the body.

1 oz. Protein (dry) = 120 C. --about 113 in the body.

1 oz. Carbohydrates (dry) = 120 C. --about 113 in the body.

Can you see now why fats are valuable? Why they make fat more than any other food? They give off more than two and one-fourth times as much heat, or energy, as the other foods.

Notice that protein and carbohydrates have the same food value as to heat or energy, each 113 Calories to the dry ounce. However, they are not interchangeable; that is, carbohydrates will not take the place of protein It is absolutely necessary to build and repair tissue, and carbohydrates cannot do that. But fats and carbohydrates are interchangeable as fuel or energy foods.

Calories Needed per Day for Normal Individuals

This depends upon age, weight, and physical activities; the baby and the growing child needing many more calories per pound per day than the adult, who has to supply only his energy and repair needs. The older adults require still less than the young adult. As to weight; I have told you why overweight individuals need so little. As to physical activities; the more active, obviously the more calories needed, for every movement consumes calories.

The Canadian lumberjack, for instance, while working during the winter months, consume from 5000 to 8000 Calories per day. But they do a tremendous amount of physical work.

Mental work does not require added nourishment. This has been proved, and if an excess be taken over what is needed at rest (if considerable exercise is not taken while doing the mental work) the work is not so well done.

Per pound per day

Child 2-6 1000 to 1600 Cal. per day Child 6-12 1600 to 2500 Cal. per day Youth 12-18 2500 to 3000 Cal. per day

(Remember that in general the boy needs as much as his father, and the girl as much as her mother.)

MAN (per day):

At rest 1800 to 2000 C. Sedentary 2200 to 2800 C. Working 3500 to 4000 C.

WOMAN (per day):

At rest 1600 to 1800 C. Sedentary occupations (bookkeeper, etc.) 2000 to 2200

C. Occupations involving standing, walking, or manual labor (general housekeeping, etc.) 2200 to 2500 C. Occupations requiring strength (factory worker, etc.) 2500 to 3000 C. (ROSE.)

Example of Finding Number of Calories Needed

1. Determine normal weight by rule.

2. Multiply normal weight by number of calories needed per pound per day.

For example, say you weigh 125 lbs., but by the rule for your height your weight should be 150 lbs.; then 150 would be the number you would use.

By the rule I have given, adults require 15-20 Calories per pound per day, depending upon activity. For example, if you have no physical activities, then take the lowest figure, 15. 150x15--2250. Therefore your requirement, if your weight should be 150, is 2250 Calories per day.

Now, if you want to lose, cut down 500-1000 Calories per day from that. Remember calories in calories him out.

Five hundred Calories equal approximately 2 ounces of fat. Two ounces per day would be about 4 pounds per month, or 48 pounds per year. Cutting out 1000 Calories per day would equal a reduction of approximately 8 pounds per month, or 96 pounds per year. These pounds you can absolutely lose by having a knowledge of food values (calories) and regulating your intake accordingly. You can now see the importance of a knowledge of calories.

Review

1. Define Calorie, and tell how determined.

2. How many C. in 1 oz. fat? of carbohydrates? of protein?

3. Why are fats so fattening?

4. How many C. per day do you require? do mental workers?

5. Upon what do C. needed per day for normal individuals depend? Discuss.

3

Review and More Definitions

FOOD: That which taken into the body builds and repairs tissue and yields energy in heat and muscular power.

CLASSES OF FOOD:

1. Protein, 18% of body weight. 2. Fats, 16% of body weight. 3. Carbohydrates, 1% of body weight. 4. Mineral matter, 5% of body weight. 5. Vitamins. 6. Water, 60% of body weight.

PROTEIN: Builds tissue, repairs waste, yields energy, and may help store fat. One-half, at least, of your protein should be from the vegetable kingdom.

A large percentage of protein is contained in

Eggs Meat Fowl Fish Nuts Milk Cheese Gluten of Wheat Legumes (beans, peas, lentils, peanuts, etc.)

There is about one-fourth ounce protein in

1 egg 1 glass milk (skim, butter, or whole) 1-1/2 oz. lean meat, or fish or fowl 1 oz. (1-1/5 cu. in.) whole milk cheese 2 slices of bread, 3-1/2 x 3-1/2 x 1/2 (white, whole wheat, corn, etc.) 3 heaping tablespoonfuls canned baked beans or Lima beans 17 peanuts

255 C. Per Oz.

FATS: Yield energy and are stored as fat.

Animal Fat: Cream, Butter, Lard

Oils: Cottonseed, Olive Almonds, Peanuts, Walnuts Chocolate, etc.

113 C. Per Oz.

CARBOHYDRATES: Yield energy and are stored as fat.

Sugars (candy, honey, syrup, sweet fruits)

Starches (breads, cereals, potatoes, corn, legumes, nuts)

Vegetable fiber, or cellulose

MINERAL MATTER: Shares in forming bones and teeth, and is necessary for proper functioning.

Carbon Lime Sodium Potassium, Sulfur Iron Phosphorus Etc.

Whole Grain Products Not Devitalized

These elements are contained largely in the outer coatings of grains, fruits, and vegetables, and in animal foods and their products. Do not pare potatoes before cooking. Cook vegetables in a small amount of water, saving the water for soups and sauces.

WATER: The universal solvent, absolutely necessary for life.

Contained in purest form in all vegetables and fruits. The average person needs, in addition, from three to five pints taken as a drink. If not sure of the purity, boil. Do not drink while food is in the mouth. Drink approximately half hour before you have a meal it will increase your digestion.

Absolutely Necessary for Growth

VITAMINES: Health preservers. Vital substances necessary for growth. The chemistry of these products is at present not thoroughly understood, but their importance has been demonstrated by experiments (not torture) on animals. By this work we know that diseases like beri-beri, scurvy, rickets, and probably pellagra, are due to a lack of these vital elements in the food, and from that fact these are called "deficiency" diseases.

It has been found that the vitamins, like the minerals, are most abundant in the outer coverings and the germ of grains, and in fruits and vegetables. They are also present in fresh milk, butter, meat and eggs. Babies fed pasteurized or boiled milk should have fruit juices and vegetable purees early. Begin with one-half teaspoonful, well diluted, and gradually increase the feeding to an ounce or more between meals once or twice daily. Babies drinking cow's milk is creating a cross species problem. Babies should only drink their mother's milk. This will eliminate earaches and respiratory illnesses.

Most animal fats have the vitamins, but vegetable fats are deficient in them. That is the reason cod liver oil is better for some therapeutic uses than olive oil.

BALANCED DIET: Should contain

10-15% Protein (children may need more) 25-30% Fat 60-65% Carbohydrates

For example, suppose you are a fairly active woman and need 2500 calories per day. Then for a balanced diet you would need:

10% Protein, or 250 C. 25% Fat, or 625 C. 65% Carbohydrates 1625 C. ------- 2500 C.

250 C. of P. = 2-1/5 oz. dry protein (250 ÷ 113 = 2-1/5, approximately) 625 C. of F. = 2-1/2 oz. of fat (625 ÷ 255 = 2-1/2, approximately) 1625 C. of CH. = 14-1/2 oz. dry carbohydrates (1625 ÷ 113 = 14-1/2, approximately)

Two and one-fifth ounces dry protein equals the approximate amount of protein in 10 ounces lean meat, fish, or fowl, or 9 ounces cheese, or 9 eggs. (You should not take all of your proteins in any of these single forms.) Two and one-half ounces fat equals approximately 5 pats of butter.

But listen! You don't have to bother with all this fussy stuff. *Be careful not to over- or under-eat of the proteins*, and your tastes will be a fair standard for the rest. You should remember that a balanced diet contains some of all these foods, in about the proportions given, and that, while *watery vegetables and fruits contain very few calories, they contain very important mineral salts, vitamins, and cellulose.* The latter is good for the daily scrub of the intestinal tract.

CONSTIPATION is many times caused by a too concentrated diet, or one containing too little roughage. It has also been discovered that some individuals who are troubled with faulty elimination digest this cellulose, and only the more resistant, like bran, is not absorbed. For those, the Japanese seaweed called agar-agar in the laboratory, but more familiarly known as agar by the layman, is excellent. The most industrious digestive tract apparently can not digest that. It has the further property of absorbing a large amount of water, thus increasing its bulk.

Mineral oils (refined paraffin) also are not absorb-able, and they act with benefit in some cases. About the worst thing to do, in general, is to take physics constantly. These are not physics, however; they act mechanically. Even the C.S. (common-sense?) individual can take these. The agar may be taken two or three heaping teaspoonfuls in a large glass of water before retiring, or in the morning before breakfast, or in lieu of 4 o'clock tea. Drink it down rapidly--for goodness' sake, don't try to chew it.

Mineral oil will make fine mayonnaise dressing. It has little or no food value, so the constipated overweight individual may indulge freely. For faulty elimination, then--

1. Correct diet.

2. Exercise--especially brisk walking. Walking will massage the intestines.

3. Regularity of habit.

4. Possibly the addition of bran, agar, or mineral oils.

5. Sweet disposition. As a side note Mean people are always constipated.

Review

1. Give classes of food, with examples of each.

2. What are vitamins? How importance discovered?

3. Where most abundant?

4. What is a balanced diet?

5. What should be done for faulty elimination?

4

More Keys and More Calories

The following list probably does not contain all of the foods you might like and want to know about, but from those named you can judge of the food value of others. In general, the caloric value, and therefore the fattening value, depends upon the amount of fat and the degree of concentration.

But remember this point: *Any food eaten beyond what your system requires for its energy, growth, and repair, is fattening, or is an irritant, or both.*

If a food contains much fat, you will know that it is high in food value, for fat has two and one-quarter times the caloric value that proteins and carbohydrates have. Dry foods are high in value, for they are concentrated and contain little water. Compare the quantity of two heaping teaspoonfuls of sugar, a concentrated food, and one and one-half pounds of lettuce, a watery vegetable, each having the same caloric value. A moderate sized chocolate cream is not only concentrated but has considerable fat in the chocolate.

It is not necessary to know accurately the caloric values. In fact, authorities differ in some of their computations. The list is not mathematically correct, but it will give you a good idea of the relative values, and is accurate enough for our purposes. I have purposely given round numbers, where possible, in order to make them more easily remembered.

In reckoning made dishes, such as puddings and sauces, you must compute the different ingredients approximately. About how much sugar it has, how much fat to the dish, and so on. In reckoning any food, if you are reducing, give it the benefit of the doubt on the high count; and if trying to gain, count it low.

It is well, if you are much overweight or underweight, to have some of these foods that are given weighed, so that you can judge approximately what your servings will total.

A mixture of foods should be used, in order to get the different elements which are necessary for the human machine. It is not wholesome to have many foods at a meal; but the menu should be varied from day to day.

Any regimen which does not allow some carbohydrates and fats for the fuel foods is injurious if persisted in for a length of time.

As to harmful combinations; there are not many, and if your food is thoroughly masticated you need not concern yourself very much about them. However, if you find a food disagrees with you, or that certain combinations disagree, do not try to use them. Underweight individuals sometimes have to train their digestive tracts for some of the foods they need.

Coffee, tea and other mild stimulants are not harmful to the majority; but, like everything else, in excess they will cause ill health. Alcoholic drinks make the fat fatter and the thin thinner, and both more feeble mentally.

There are many books which go into the subject much more deeply." The Home Dietitian," written by , Dr. Belle Wood-Com stock

"Feeding the Family," by Mary Schwartz Rose, and "Dietary Computer," by Pope. There are doubtless many other good ones. .

Measuring Table

1 teaspoon (tsp.) fluid 1/6 oz. 1 dessertspoon (tsp.) 1/3 oz. 1 tablespoon (tbsp.) 1/2 oz. 1 ordinary cup 8 oz. 1 ordinary glass 8 oz. Average helping a.h.

One Hundred Calorie Portions and Average Helpings

(Approximate Measures)

MEATS

Beefsteak, lean round.................................2 oz. 100 C. A.h....... 3-1/2 oz., 185 C.

Beefsteak, tenderloin..................................1 oz. 100 C. A.h.................. 285 C.

Beef, roast, very lean...................................3 oz. 100 C. A.h.................. 150 C.

Chicken, roast...1-2/3oz. 100 C. 1 slice.............. 180 C.

Frankfurters, 1 sausage.............................1 oz. 100 C.

Chops, lamb or mutton...................1-1/2 oz. 100 C. Average chops.... 150-300 C.

Pork: Bacon, crisp.......................................1/2 oz. 100 C. 1 small slice, crisp 25 C.

Chop.....................................1-1/2 oz. 100 C. Medium..........160-300 C.

Ham, boiled...1-1/3 oz. 100 C. A.h..........3 oz., 250 C.

Ham, fried...3/4 oz. 100 C. A.h..........3 oz., 400 C.

Sausage.......................................1 oz. 100 C. 1 small, crisp.......60 C.

Turkey...1-1/3 oz. 100 C. A.h........3-1/3 oz., 260 C.

Fish Boiled or Broiled

FISH

Fish, Lean, Cod, Halibut..............................3 oz. 100 C. A.h........... 4 oz., 135 C.

Fish, fat, salmon, sardines ....1 1/2 oz. 100 C. A.h........... 4 oz., 260 C.

Lobster...4 oz. 100 C. A.h................. 100 C.

Oysters... 12 100 C. 1 oyster.............. 8 C.

Clams, long.. 8 100 C. 1 clam............... 12 C.

SOUPS

Cream soups, average.................................3 oz. 100 C. A.h........... 4 oz., 125 C.

Consomme, no fat......................................30 oz. 100 C. A.h........... 4 oz., 15 C.

DAIRY PRODUCTS AND EGGS

Butter, 1 level tbsp. Scant .... 1/2 oz. 100 C. 1 ball.............. 120 C.

Cheese (American, Roquefort, Swiss, etc.)................. 1-1/8 cu. in 3/4 oz. 100 C.

Cottage Cheese.. 3 oz. 100 C. A.h................. 100 C.

Whole Milk.. 5 oz. 100 C. 1 glass............. 160 C.

Skim Milk.. 10 oz. 100 C. 1 glass............. 80 C.

Malted Milk (dry)...1 h. tbsp. 100 C.

Buttermilk, natural.. 10 oz. 100 C. 1 glass............. 80 C.

Koumiss.. 6 oz. 100 C. 1 glass............ 130 C.

Condensed, unsweetened........................... 2 oz. 100 C. 1 tbsp............... 35 C.

Condensed, sweetened, ...1-1/4 tbsp....... 100 C.

Cream, average...1-1/3 oz. 100 C. 1 tbsp............... 50 C.

Cream, whipped..................................... 1-1/3 oz. 100 C. 1 h. tbsp........... 100 C.

Eggs, 1 large.. 1 100 C. Average egg........... 80 C.

Boiled or poached; if fried, C. depend upon fat adhering.

VEGETABLES

When not otherwise indicated, the method of cooking is by boiling. The caloric value of sauces served with them not included.

Asparagus, large stalks.. 20 100 C. 1 stalk................ 5 C.

Beets.. 1 lb. 100 C. 2 h. tbsp............ 30 C.

Beans, Baked, home...............................1-1/2 oz. 100 C. 3 h. tbsp........... 300 C.

Beans, Baked, canned...........................2-1/2 oz. 100 C. 3 h. tbsp........... 150 C.

Beans, Lima.. 3 oz. 100 C. 3 h. tbsp........... 130 C.

Beans, String.. 1 lb. 100 C. 2 h. tbsp............ 15 C.

Cabbage.. 1-1/2 lb. 100 C. 3 h. tbsp............. 10 C.

Carrots.. 1 lb. 100 C. 3 h. tbsp............. 20 C.

Cauliflower... 1 lb. 100 C. 3 h. tbsp............. 20 C.

Celery, uncooked... 1 lb. 100 C. 6 stalks............. 15 C.

Corn, canned... 3-1/3 oz. 100 C. 2 h. tbsp............ 100 C.

Corn, green, 1 ear.................................... 3-1/3 oz. 100 C. Medium size.

Cucumber.. 1-1/2 lb. 100 C. 10 to 12 thin slices.. 10 C.

Lettuce... 1-1/2 lb. 100 C. A.h................. 5-10 C.

Mushrooms.. 8 oz. 100 C.

Onions, 2 large... 8 oz. 100 C.

Parsnips....................................... 8 oz. 100 C. A.h............ 2 oz., 25 C.

Peas, green....................................... 3 oz. 100 C. A.h., 3 h. tbsp...... 100 C.

Potatoes, sweet.................................. 1-1/2 oz. 100 C. 1 medium............. 200 C.

Potatoes, white... 3 oz. 100 C. 1 medium............ 100 C.

Potato Chips......scant................................ 1 oz. 100 C. A.h., 8-10 pieces.... 100 C.

Radishes... 1 lb. 100 C. A.h., 6 red button.... 15 C.

Spinach.................................... 1-1/2 lb. 100 C. A.h., 1/2 cup......... 25 C.

Squash.................................... 1 lb. 100 C. A.h., 2h. tbsp........ 25 C.

Tomatoes.................................... 1 lb. 100 C. A.h., 1 large......... 50 C.

Turnips.. 1 lb. 100 C. A.h., 2 h. tbsp....... 25 C.

FRUITS

Apple....................................... 7 oz. 100 C. 1 average size......... 50 C.

Banana...................................... 5 oz. 100 C. 1 small.............. 100 C.

Berries............average........................... 5 oz. 100 C. 1 small cup.......... 100 C.

Cantaloupe............................... 1 lb. 100 C. A.h., 1/2 melon....... 100 C.

Cherries.................................... 5 oz. 100 C. A.h., 1 small cup..... 100 C.

Grapes.. 5 oz. 100 C. A.h., 1 small bunch... 100 C.

Lemons (5 oz. Each)........................ 2 100 C. They won't make you thin. Average
....size........... 30 C.

Oranges (9 oz. Each)............................... 1 100 C.

Peaches (5 oz. Each)............................... 2 100 C. Average size........... 50 C.

Pears (6 oz. Each)................................. 1 100 C. Average size........... 90 C.

Pineapple, fresh.................................... 7 oz. 100 C. 2 slices, 1 in. thick. 100 C.

Plums, large................................. 3 or 4 100 C. 1 plum................. 30 C.

Watermelon............................. 1-1/2 lb. 100 C. Large slice........... 15 C.

Dates (dry), large................................ 3-4 100 C. 1 large............... 25 C.

Figs (dry), large................................ 1-1/2 100 C. 1 large............... 65 C.

Prunes (dry), large................................ 3 100 C. 1 large............... 35 C.

Stewed, 4 medium, with 4 tbsp. Juice.................... 200 C.

BREAD AND CRACKERS

Brown Bread, 1 slice, 3 in. in dial., 3/4 in. thick 100 C.

Corn Bread, 3 x 2 x 3/4 1-1/2 oz. 100 C.

Victory Bread, 1 slice, 3 x 4 x 1/2 in. 100 C.

White, gluten, rye, whole wheat, etc., practically same caloric value per same
weight. There is so little difference between the caloric value of gluten bread and
other breads that it is not necessary for reducing to try to get it. (Toasted bread
has the same caloric value that it had before toasting. It is more easily digested,
but just as fattening. Advised, however, because it makes you chew.)

1 French or Vienna roll 100 C.

Zwieback 3/4 oz. 100 C. 1 slice, 3-1/4 x 1-1/4 x 1/2 in., 35 C.

Graham Crackers 3 100 C. 1 c., 3 in. sq. 35 C.

Oyster Crackers 24 100 C. Soda Crackers 4 100 C. 1 c. 25 C.

Pretzels 5 100 C. 1 p. 20 C.

BREAKFAST FOODS, ETC.

Farina or Cream of Wheat 6 oz. 100 C. 2 h. tbsp 60 C. Force 1 oz. 100 C. 5 h. tbsp 65 C.

Grape nuts scant 1 oz. 100 C. 2 tbsp 100 C.

Griddle Cakes, 4-1/2 in. in diam 100 C. A.h., 3 cakes 300 C. (This does not include butter and syrup, remember.)

Hominy 4 oz. 100 C. 2 h. tbsp 85 C.

Macaroni, plain 4 oz. 100 C. 2 h. tbsp 90 C.

Macaroni and cheese (depends on amt. cheese) 2 h. tbsp 200-300 C.

Muffin, average 3/4 m. 100 C. 1 muffin 125 C.

Oatmeal 5 oz. 100 C. 1 small cup 100 C.

Puffed Rice 1 oz. 100 C. 5 h. tbsp 50 C.

Popcorn (cups) 1-1/2 100 C. A.h. depends on butter added.

Rice, boiled 4 oz. 100 C. 1/2 cup 100 C.

Shredded Wheat Biscuit 1 100 C. Triscuits (2) 100 C. Waffles scant 1/2 w. 100 C. 1 waffle 225 C.

CANDY, PASTRIES AND SWEETS

Chocolate creams, medium. 1 100 C.

Chocolate, 1 lb 2880 C.

Cherries, candied 10 100 C.

Cup Custard, 1/3 cup 100 C.

Chocolate Nut Caramels 1 x 1 x 4/5 in. 100 C.

Other candies, reckon sugar, nuts, etc.

Cookies, plain, diam 3 in. 2 100 C. 1 cookie 50 C. If raisins or nuts in them, count extra.

Doughnut scant 2/3 100 C. 1 average size 160 C.

Ginger-snap 5 100 C. 1 gingersnap 20 C.

Honey h. tbsp. 1 100 C. Thick syrups approximately the same.

Ladyfingers scant 1 oz. 100 C. 1 ladyfinger 35-50 C.

Macaroons 2 100 C. 1 macaroon 50 C.

Pie with top crust, about 1/4 ordinary slice, or 1-1/4 in. 100 C. A.h., 1/6 pie 350 C.

Pie without top crust, 2 in. 100 C.

Custard, lemon, squash, etc. A.h., 1/6 pie. 250-300 C.

Puddings, average cup 1/4 100 C. A.h. 200-350 C. Depends upon richness.

Ice Cream h. tbsp. 1 100 C. A.h. 200-350 C. Depends upon richness.

Cakes 1 oz. 100 C. A.h. 200-350 C. Depends upon size, icing, fruit, nuts, etc.; compute approximately. Sugar cubes 3 100 C. Granulated h. tsp. 2 100 C.

Saccharine, a coal tar product 300 to 500 times sweeter than sugar, but of no food value. Not advisable to use habitually. Better learn to like things unsweetened--it can be done.

CONDIMENTS AND SAUCES

Mayonnaise m. tbsp. 1 100 C. A.h. 200 C.

Olive oil and other oils. dsp. 1 100 C.

Olives, green or ripe 6-8 100 C. 1 olive 10-15 C.

Tomato Catchup 6 oz. 100 C. 1 tbsp. 10 C. Thick Gravies tbsp. 3 100 C.

NUTS

Almonds, large 10 100 C. 1 almond 10 C.

Brazil, large 2-1/2 100 C. 1 Brazil nut 45 C.

Chestnuts, small 20 100 C. 1 chestnut 5 C.

Peanuts, large double 10 100 C. 1 bag 250-300 C.

Pecans, large 5 100 C. 1 pecan 20 C.

Walnuts, large 3-1/3 100 C. 1 walnut 30 C.

Cocoanut, prepared 1/2 oz. 100 C. Peanut Butter 2-1/2 tsp. 100 C.

If you will remember the following portions of food, you will have a standard by which to compute your servings:

Lean Meat: a piece 3 x 2 x 1/2 (2 oz.) 100 C.

Now if your serving of meat or fish is fat, mentally cut in two for same value. If very lean, you should add a little.

White Bread: slice 3 x 4x 1/2 100 C. Compute other breads by this.

Butter: 1 scant tablespoonful 100 C.

Sugar: 1 heaping teaspoonful 50 C.

Potatoes: 1 medium, boiled or baked. 100 C.

Watery Vegetables: 1 helping 15-35 C.

If food is fried, or butter, oil, or cream sauces are added, the C. value increases markedly.

Review

1. Why is a mixture of foods necessary?

2. Give the caloric value of the following: 1 glass of milk, skim; buttermilk; 10 chocolate creams; 1 bag peanuts; 1 pat butter; 1 piece pie.

3. Name foods low in caloric value. Why are they valuable?

4. How many calories of bread and butter do you daily consume?

5. Reckon your usual caloric intake. How much of it is in excess of your needs?

6. Memorize caloric value of foods you are fond of.

This Table of Foods, With the C Given Per Oz. Will Help You

The caloric value of pure fat is 255 C per oz., dry starches and sugars (carbohydrates), and protein (the meat element), is 113. This means fats are 2-1/4 times more fattening than other foods. Most foods contain considerable water, so the following is an approximate table of foods 'as is.' I have given round numbers in the table so you can more easily remember them. *Memorize it.*

Calories per oz.

Fats 255 Nuts, edible part 200 Sugar 115 Cream cheese 110 Cottage cheese (no fat) 30 Breads 75 Lean meats 50 Lean fish 35 Eggs (per oz.) 40 Milk, whole 20 Milk, skim and buttermilk (no fat) 10 Milk, condensed, sweet 100 Milk, condensed, unsweetened 50 Cream, thin 60 Cream, thick 110 Fruits: Dried 100 Sweet 25 Acid 15 Vegetables: Potatoes, plain (oz.) 30 Cooked Legumes, (peas, beans, etc.) 20-35 Watery and leafy 5-15

5

Vegetarianism vs. Meat Eating

As protein is the only food which builds and repairs tissue, it is the food which has caused the most controversy.

First: As to the amount needed.

Second: As to whether animal flesh protein is necessary.

AMOUNT NEEDED: It was thought for many years that 150 grams or 5 ounces of dry protein (equivalent to about 1-1/2 pounds lean meat) per day was necessary. But experiments of Chittenden and others have proved that considerably less is sufficient, and that the health is improved if less is taken.

Chittenden's standard is 50 grams, or 1-2/3 ounces, dry protein (equivalent to 1/2 pound meat per day). This is considered by many as insufficient. A variation from 1-2/3 to 3 ounces dry protein per day will give a safe range. (ROSE.)

Approx. 240 to 360 C Per Day

The amount of protein needed is comparatively independent of the amount of physical exertion, thus differing from the purely fuel foods, carbohydrates and fats, which should vary in direct proportion to the amount of physical exertion. In general, 10 to 15 per cent of the total calories per day should be taken as protein. An excess is undoubtedly irritant to the kidneys, blood vessels, and other organs, and if too little is taken the body tissues will suffer.

Not all of the protein should be taken in the form of animal protein; at least one-half should be taken from the vegetable kingdom.

Animal Flesh Protein

The following are a few of the chief reasons given by those who object to its use:

First: The animal has just as much right to life, liberty, and pursuit of happiness as we have.

Second: They may be diseased, and there is the possibility of their containing animal parasites, such as tapeworms and trichina. I would like to tell you more about worms, they are so interesting, but He says not to try to tell all I know in this little book; that maybe he will let me write another sometime, although it is a terrible strain on him, and that I have given enough of the family history, anyway.

Third: The tissues of animals contain excremental material, which may cause excess acidity, raise the blood pressure, and so forth.

Fourth: More apt to purify and thus give ptomaine poisoning.

Fifth: Makes the disposition more vicious.

(Honest,--animals eating meat exclusively are more vicious.)

Those who believe that animal protein should be eaten answer these points as follows:

First: Survival of the fittest.

Second: If you give decent support to your health departments they can furnish enough inspectors to prevent the marketing of diseased meat; and if some should slip through, if you thoroughly bake, boil, or fry your animal parasites they will lose their pep.

Third: Most of the harmful products are destroyed by the intestines and liver.

Fourth: True, but see that you get good meat, and don't eat it in excess.

Fifth: Unanswerable--to be proved later by personal experiments.

In addition, they say that animal protein is more easily digested, that 97 per cent is assimilated because it is animal, and so it is much more to be desired, especially by children and convalescents; that vegetable protein is enclosed in cellulose, and only 65 to 75 per cent is used by the system; thus the diet is apt to be too bulky if the proper amount is taken.

It has been proved, however, by several endurance tests, that the vegetarian contestants had more strength and greater endurance than their meat-eating competitors, so there is no reason why we should be worried by one or two, or even more, meatless days, especially when animal product protein, such as milk, eggs, cheese, and the vegetable proteins, as in the legumes and the nuts, are available.

Protein Calories in 100 C Portions of Food

In 100 C's Bread, 1 slice, (W.W. the highest) 12 to 16 C's P In 100 C's

Cooked Cereals, 1 Sm cup, (oatmeal highest) 10 to 18 C's P In 100 C's

Rice, 1 small cup 10 C's P In 100 C's

Macaroni, 1 small cup 15 C's P In 100 C's

Whole milk, 5 oz. 20 C's P In 100 C's

Skim and buttermilk, 10 oz. 35 C's P In 100 C's

Cheese, 3 heaping tbsp. Cottage cheese 75 C's P In 100 C's

Eggs 1-1/3 36 C's P In 100 C's

Meat or fish, Very lean 2-3 oz. 50 to 75 C's P In 100 C's

Nuts, peanuts, almonds, walnuts. Peanuts the highest 10 to 20 C's P In 100 C's

Beans 1/3 cup average 20 C's P In 100 C's

Green peas 3/4 cup average 28 C's P In 100 C's

Corn 1/3 cup average 12 C's P In 100 C's

Onions 3 to 4 medium 12 C's P In 100 C's

Potato 1 medium 12 C's P In 100 C's Tomatoes 1 lb 15 C's P In 100 C's

Fresh fruits: berries, currants, rhubarb 10 C's P Others 2 to 5 C's P

6

The Deluded Ones--My Thin Friends

When you worry needlessly, notice how tense your muscles are. You are exercising them all of the time and using hundreds of calories of energy. You raise your blood pressure, the internal secreter glands may overact (re-read what I have said about these glands in the fat people), and thus many more calories are used. The intestinal secretions do not flow so freely, you have indigestion and do not assimilate your food, and thus hundreds more calories are lost.

It certainly is impossible to gain unless your food is assimilated.

So the first thing you have to learn is this mental control and to relax. Remember that word, relax. After you are better nourished your nervous system will not be on hair-trigger tension, and it will be easier for you.

If you are ill in mind or body, remember that it is natural to be well, and that within your body nature has stored the most wonderful forces which are always tending towards the normal, or health, if not obstructed or hindered.

Nature sometimes needs help to stimulate those forces, or to reinforce them, or to remove obstructions. This is where the physician comes in. But you yourself can aid nature the most by realizing that *nature is health and it is normal to be well*. By so doing, all of your organs function better and you are restored to normal more rapidly.

Second: It is very important to have enough sleep. Dr. Richard Cabot says that probably resistance is lowered as much by lack of sufficient sleep as by any other factor, and that all you can soak into your system in twenty-four hours is not too much. Don't forget the fresh air.

You generally suffer from sleeplessness, I believe. The overweight's are always advised not to sleep too much. They will find while reducing that they won't want to sleep so much, anyway. They will like to stay awake--they feel so much happier.

Now, when you retire and try to sleep but cannot, try this--it works with me. You know when you are passing over your mental images become distorted and grotesque. I artificially induce that state. If I find myself rehearsing about two hundred times, with appropriate gestures, the keen, witty, logical remarks which I could have made in favor of my pet legislation in the club discussion, but didn't, then I begin after this fashion:

Pink elephants with green ribbons on their tails--red rhinoceros (is that right, or should it be rhinoceroses?)--smiling peanuts--Woman's City Club--Social Health Insurance--why didn't I say--I wish I had said--(here get out, you annoyance!)--pink elephants--and so forth and so forth.

Now I realize I have ruined myself. I am my own worst enemy. I have exposed my whole life before those modern vivisectionists, the army of amateur psycho-analysts.

Third: Exercise. Great muscular exertion should be avoided, but the setting-up exercises that I advise, if begun with moderation and increased gradually, will undoubtedly stimulate the appetite and help the body functions to be better performed.

Fourth: Since food is the only source of body substance, you must gradually train your stomach so that it can care for enough food to not only supply your bodily energy, but to leave a little excess to be stored as fat.

If you have a small appetite--and many of you have--your stomach is undoubtedly contracted, and you must gradually add to the amount you have been eating, even though it may cause some distress, until you have disciplined it so that it can handle what you need without distress. The stomach is a muscular organ and can be trained and exercised somewhat as other organs can. You will not have much appetite at first, but it will develop. Sometimes a short fast for a day or two, drinking nothing but pure water, seems to be beneficial in the beginning.

Do not drink much with your meals, unless the drink has food value by the addition of lots of cream or sugar, or both.

Decide how many calories you need for your activities, gradually add to your dietary until you have reached that number, and then some more, and you will gain as surely as the overweight individual will lose by doing the opposite. It may take a long time, or you may get results very rapidly, depending somewhat upon the individual characteristics. Gradually increase your butter, cream, sugar, chocolate, and so forth, as they are very high in food value.

Study the Key to the Calories and reckon your calories every day for a while. You have already noticed that the foods that you like are low in food value.

Here are some of the things you can take to add to your fuel:

A glass of milk, hot or cold, taken between meals and before retiring, will add about 500 calories.

Cream sauce on your vegetables will add to their value.

Cod liver oil, or olive oil, or cream, begun in small doses and gradually increased.

One malted milk, made with milk, syrup, egg, ice cream, whipped cream, and the malted milk, will add about 500 calories.

You remember the painful time that I spoke of when there was so much more of me than there ought to be? Well, the aforesaid concoction, made with milk, syrup, egg, ice cream, whipped cream, and the malted milk, was an accessory before the fact, and also particeps criminis before the law.

I absorbed this phraseology by doing much research of the several weight loss organizations and Professional Women's Clubs, like the ones below with their high-class women attorneys, ministers, dentists, Ph. D's, and "Medical Trust" doctors.

"Medical Trust."--The American Medical Association (A.M.A.), a powerful trust you can't get into unless you have a high preliminary education and are a graduate of a high-class medical college. Eleven years' training after the grammar school is their minimum standard now.

"League for Medical Ignorance."--The so-called "League for Medical Freedom"; the opponent of the above mentioned trust. Their standard--any old kind of a medical or religious training, two weeks or longer, or just anyone who has the money to pay for the course. No education, no barrier; in fact, those of limited education make the loudest boosters for the league. In justice, I must say that many splendid, estimable persons belong to this league, not knowing these facts.

Also have your teeth X-rayed. Blind abscesses at the roots will cause all sorts of aches and pains, as well as underweight.

Sixth: *Don't talk so much.* See if you can't leave out two-thirds of the totally unimportant, uninteresting details. A tremendous amount of energy is used in talking. This habit I would not say was confined to you, by any means; it is another one of those pretty nearly universal errors.

I will not give you a sample fattening menu, for it might be all out of proportion to what you could handle, and it would upset you. Make out your own menus, realizing that you must work gradually to the desired amount.

I am taking it for granted that you are organically sound, that your scientific, educated physician has said there is nothing the matter with you, except perhaps your "nervous" disposition.

Have I not been nice to you? All right, relax and watch yourself get into the class of the plump and more than adequate in weight.

And if you don't succeed after a faithful trial, take the milk-cure, with its three to six weeks' absolute rest.

Recapitulation

1. Calm yourself. 2. Sleep. 3. Exercise. 4. Food. 5. Masticate 6. Delete the details. 7. Milk-cure.

Review

1. Repeat Elbert Hubbard's advice. 2. Give three reasons why worry can make you thin. 3. Define "Medical Trust" and "League for Medical Freedom." 4. Memorize paragraph about nature 5. Enumerate the things you can eat to increase your calories.

On the next few pages is something I found on the internet. The author is unknown but it speaks volumes.

4.2 grams = 1 teaspoon of sugar = 1 cube !
Someone ought to get an award for this. *We know*
the facts, but this
brings it into perspective quickly, doesn't it?
Each cube is a teaspoonful.

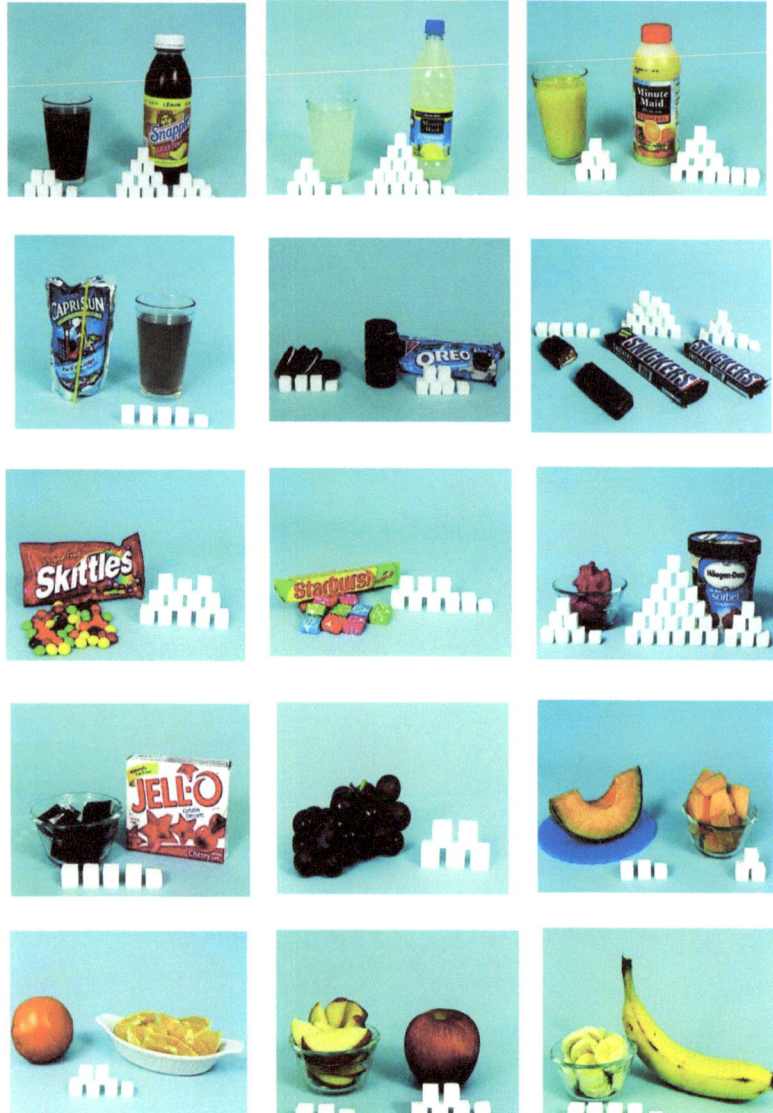

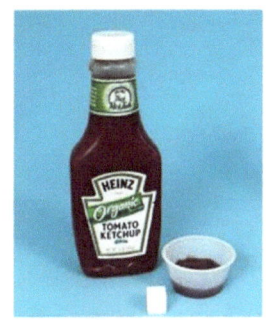

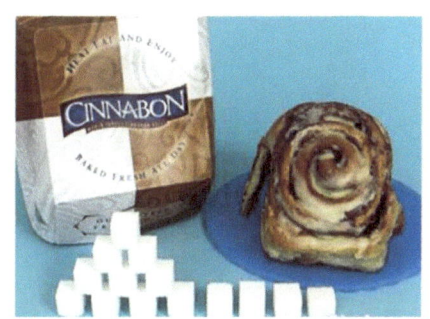

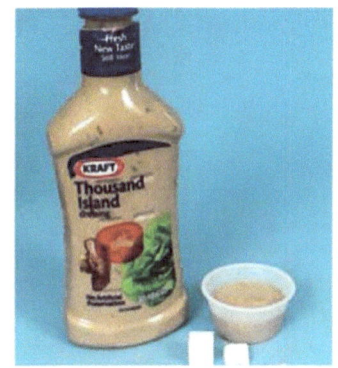

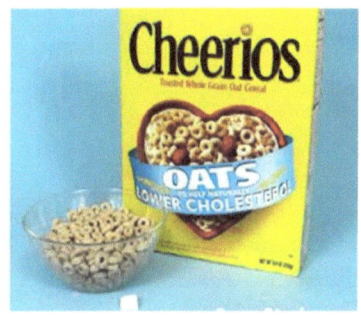

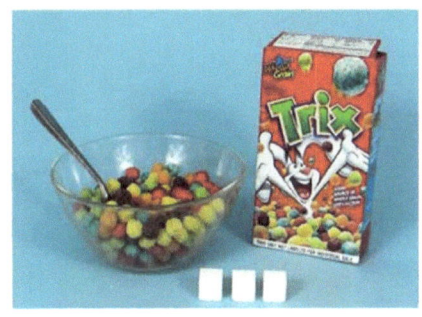

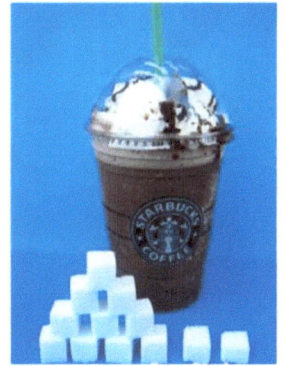

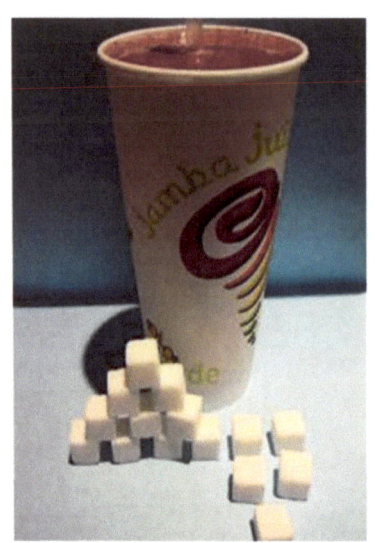
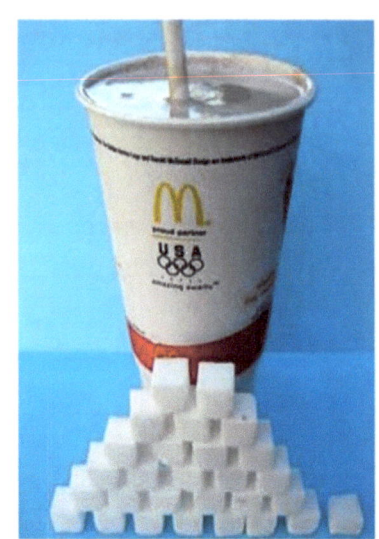

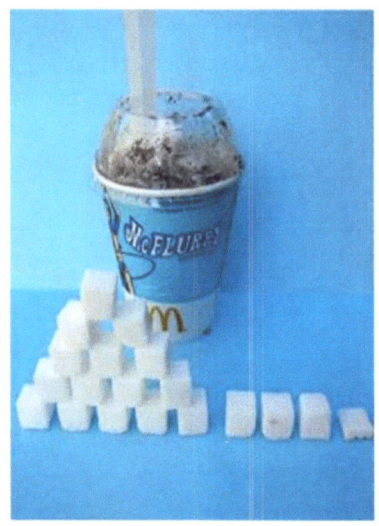

as they say: A picture is worth a thousand words.

Exercise

It is practically impossible to reduce weight through exercise alone, unless one can do a tremendous amount of it. For the food that one eats is usually enough to cover the energy lost by the exercise. As I've stated several times in this book hypnotherapy, proper dieting and exercise is the combination needed to lose weight. Hypnotherapy will eliminate hunger pangs are the desire for the food, the proper dieting or food intake will eliminate the calories and the exercise will cause you to burn more calories which in turn will always will help you lose weight.

However, exercise is a very important feature of any reducing program; not because of the fat that is burned up in the exercise--and there is some burned--but for the reason that it is necessary to keep one in a healthy condition. The muscles, the internal organs, the bones, the brain, are all benefited--in fact, the entire system. The blood stream is cleansed by the elevation of the heart rate and the heart muscle will grow stronger. Exercise is a very important part of being healthy.

The exercises described hereinafter will help make you fat or thin, and they will keep you supple, graceful, and light on your feet.

If you have not been accustomed to exercise, I warn you to start slowly and only take up only one or two of these exercises at a time and do each one a few times only. You will be more than likely be sore, and you will realize that you have muscles in places you didn't know you had.

However sore you become, persist, if you are sure there are no organic reasons why you shouldn't--such as a weak heart. (In case you are very much overweight, I think it advisable to wait until you have reduced somewhat.) Make sure you see a physician before you start any type of exercise program that is very, very important.

It is splendid if you belong to a gym or to a physical culture class, but ten to fifteen minutes' systematic daily exercise practiced with energy, and each set followed by deep breathing, will do more good than a gym that you attend every now and then. Brisk walking with a long stride isn't so bad; in fact, if taken with a very long stride it will twist 'most every organ you have in your body. Remember, this twisting is massaging the internal organs just like chewing massages the sinuses and causes sinus drainage.

There are hundreds of exercises you can do. .

If possible, it is best to take the exercises on awaking in the morning, but if you have a job away from the home, or a household to care for you may not be able to do so. For those who have to do their own work, it may be well to do the work first. You can do it in half the time if you plan it carefully and speed up. (This advice is not for my thin friends; their speedometers register too high already.) It does not matter so much when the exercises are done as that they are done, and done every day for the rest of your life, with the possible exception of two or three days a month.

Gallstones, permanent stiff joints, and other little things like that will have a hard time forming.

My Exercises

These exercises executed with vim, and vigor--deep breathing between each set--will take ten to fifteen minutes. Re-read my warning.

1. Feet together, arms outstretched, palms up, describe as large a circle as possible. Fine for round shoulders and fat backs. Do slowly and stretch fifteen times. Smile.

2. Arms outstretched, swing to right and to left as far as possible at least 15 times each.

3. Bend sideways, to right and left, alternately, as far as possible at least 15 times each.

4. Revolve the body upon the hips from right to left at least 10 times, and left to right the same.

5. Bend and touch the floor with your fingers, without bending your knees, at least 15 times.

6. Knee-bending exercise, at least 15 times. This is hard at first.

7. Hand on door or wall, swing each leg back and forth at least 15 times. To the side 15 times. Turn head, raise arm, and tense both.

8. Step on chair with each foot at least 10 times. This is good for calf and thigh muscles. After a while you won't look as though you needed a derrick to get onto a street car.

9. Arms on sides of chair. Come down and touch abdomen. Fine for back and abdomen. Fifteen times.

Do this this for a few minutes, followed by a nice long warm bath or shower.

8

At Last! How to Reduce

The title of this chapter indicates to whom it is addressed. All others please refrain from reading, for it is strictly private and confidential, and is intended only for those who need it.

You thin and you normal people had better save it, though, for you may qualify later when you're my age. I wanted to tell my overweight friends that the first thing they have to do is to get control of their will power, and the best way to do that in my humble opinion is hypnotherapy.

Somehow, will power with a layer of fat on it gets feeble. Don't laugh! It gets worse than feeble, if there is no fat at all and the nervous system is starved, it-- well, it will slowly begin eating your muscles. So a little fat on your body is desirable but too much is a health hazard especially around the middle.

Will power, being feeble to a greater or less degree, must be bolstered and aided a bit, to begin with, so do a hypnotherapy session to bolster up your willpower so that we can get started.

First Order

Tell loudly and frequently to all your friends that you realize that it is unhealthy to be fat and that you are going to reduce to a normal weight. Let them know that you're going to hypnotherapy to lose weight. Ask them to help you by not offering you foods that will be bad for you. If you belong to a club, round up the overweight's and form a section. Call it the "Watch Your Weight--Class." Tax the members sufficiently to buy a good, accurate pair of scales. Meet once a week to weigh. Wear approximately the same weight clothes, and weigh at the same time in relation to eating. Do this whether or not you belong to a club. Once a week is often enough to weigh. Scales vary, so try to use the same ones. Remember "**weight is just a number**". *How you feel and how you look is more important than a number.*

Don't be discouraged if some day after you have eaten properly but I you seem to have gained weight. Nature sometimes seems cruel that way. The excess weight is probably due to a retention of water, and will not be permanent. However, don't depend upon this too often! Usually, if you have gained when you think you ought not to, it is because Nature has been counting calories and you haven't. I recommend that if your are going to weigh yourself weekly do it early in the morning right after you get up and take your shower. It seems that early in the morning. You actually weigh less than you do in the evenings because you're not retaining the water. If you did form that group at your gym or health club, have the members listed on a weight chart conspicuously placed near the scales, and record accurately the weight weekly.

Those not reducing at least one pound per week to be fined soundly and the proceeds given to the a local charity. That won't be a good way to raise large funds for the charity, though, for there will be no fines after the first week or so, when the members find what their maintenance diet should be and are consuming less than that.

I will explain this maintenance diet business. You shameless thin ones, call back your more polite comrades--this is important for all of you. (I shall also tell you more fully about this in the last chapter.)

The maintenance diet is one which maintains you at your present weight, *i.e.,* you are not gaining or losing. You may be over or under normal, but are staying there. The intake equals the outgo. Also reinforcement at your hypnotherapist will help your maintenance dieting beautifully.

When you eat less than your maintenance diet, you are going to supply the deficiency with your own fat.

So commit yourself on your honor that you are going to reduce or perish--no joke; you can't tell how near you are to it if you are much overweight. There are two general stages of fatty heart. In the first stage the heart is surrounded by a blanket of fat, and it also penetrates between the muscles. Later, if it goes on too long, the heart muscle itself degenerates to fat, then--

Shakespeare warns you to make thy body less, hence thy grace more; leave gormandizing, and know that the grave doth gape for thee thrice wider than for other men. Hard to understand the language, but it basically "stay slim in you dotage and you will stay healthy".

Second Order

Your stomach, long used to an excess of food for your needs--it may not be a large amount--but still, I repeat, being used to an excess of food for your needs, your stomach must be disciplined. It is undoubtedly distended, as it should not be. After a couple of days of eating properly and smaller amounts your stomach lining will begin to shrink.

A good way to show it that you are master is to fast for at least one day--drink nothing but pure water, hot or cold, as you prefer. Cold water would be the best because your body will have to heat it, thus causing you to burn calories heating the water. It will protest vociferously and will tell all its friends, the different organs of your body, how you are persecuting it, and they will join the league against you and decide they will oust you from your position, and you will feel like--but don't mind it; it will soon know that you mean business, and, much chastened and considerably contracted, will take the next day a very small amount of food very gratefully.

If you do not want to be so severe with it you can allow it five glasses of hot or cold skim milk or buttermilk, one every three hours, say, at 10,1,4,7, and 10 o'clock. One glass is 80 calories, five equal 400 calories, which is not so much.

I personally prefer once a day to have a milkshake made of 2% milk ice cubes in a protein mix that you can buy at Walmart, CVS or any other drug store and occasionally I'll put a banana in. Then I put I all that into a blender and I make about a 32 ounce drink. A drink that size obviously fills me up and I'm not hungry until it's time for my next meal.

The baked potato and glass of skim milk diet, three times a day one day a week, which has its devotees, depends upon its low caloric content for its results. There is no magic in it, no yeast business which reduces. This is most wholesome, however, for potatoes contain a large amount of the potassium salts, which tend to counteract the effects of uric acid, and thus are good mostly for the gouty type.

The beefsteak, the milk, and the fruit diets are also good. One can gain as well as lose on the milk diet, all depending on number of calories consumed, and it is an excellent method for both. The beefsteak diet is beneficial for a short time, but too much protein over a long period has been shown to be harmful. An exclusive fruit diet is excellent for reduction.

Low calorie days can be repeated once a week if necessary in order to keep the stomach in good order. Fruit juice, one-quarter glass, or fresh fruit, can be substituted for the skim milk, and you may prefer it.

You could keep on this for some time, or fast for some time, and probably be much benefited. I semi-fasted 21 days once, or rather water approximately a gallon a day, a small amount of white meat in a small amount of vegetable. I lost about twenty pounds,

It was during that period of which I have spoken, and of which I am ashamed that I should have known better. But you know that it is easier to teach twenty what should be done than to be one of twenty to follow our own teaching.

After reading about these different ways and the effects of the actions, I hope you will understand why I recommend that you start with a hypnotherapist.

Third Order

Now you will have to reckon on the amount of food or number of calories you need per day. Review the rule I have given. You find for your age and *normal weight* that you will need, let us say for example, 2200 calories. You have probably been consuming twice that amount and either storing it away as fat or as disease. (It is surprising how small an excess will gradually add up pounds of fat. For instance, three pats of butter or three medium chocolate creams a day, if over the maintenance limit, would add approximately *27 pounds a year* to your weight!)

Now you are to reduce your maintenance diet--the 2200 calories we are taking for example--to 1200 calories--quite a comfortable lot, you will find.

You will be surprised how much 1200 calories will be if the food is judiciously selected.

You may be hungry at first, but using hypnotherapy you will soon become accustomed to the change. I find that dry lemon or orange peel, or those little aromatic breath sweeteners, just a tiny bit, seem to stop the hunger pangs. I'm sure you're familiar with the fact that if you prepare the food in the kitchen you're usually not as hungry when it's time to eat. That's aromatherapy in my mind. Or you may simply have a cup of fat-free bouillon or half an apple, or other low calorie food. (Count the calories here.)

One thousand calories less food per day equals four ounces of fat lost daily-- approximately 8 pounds per month. If you do not want to lose so fast, do not cut down so much. Stay away from sodas, especially diet sodas. If you're going to drink coffee or tea. Do not add sugar. Remember that sugar adds calories and every sodas that you drink has at least 120 calories per 8 ounce bottle.

Fourth Order

You may eat just what you like--candy, pie, cake, fat meat, butter, cream--but-- *count your calories!* You can't have many nor large helpings, you see; but isn't it comforting to know that you can eat these things? Maybe some meal you would rather have a 350-calorie piece of luscious pie, with a delicious 150-calorie tablespoonful of whipped cream on it, than all of the succulent vegetables in the fridg.

My idea of heaven is a place with moist chocolate cake and whipped cream. Now that you know you can have the things you like, proceed to make your menus containing very little of them. Just remember to count the calories for each meal and make sure that the daily caloric intake is where you need to be.

Fifth Order

This is going to be your chief business and pursuit in life for the next few months, this reducing of your weight. However, keep up your training at the gym and all other activities, fast and furiously, so that you won't be thinking about yourself.

Don't reduce more than two or three pounds a week; two or less is better. If you are too cannibalistic, your heart, kidneys and nervous system are liable to suffer-- you yourself are supplying too much fat in your dietary, and there are other scientific reasons against reducing too rapidly.

I have found that the people that lose weight quickly have a tendency to regain it and more later. The key, is to change the way and the volume that you eat, not to just lose weight. In this case, less is more.

However, you may find that the first week or so you may reduce five or seven pounds; but don't worry about this, for that is a slushy, watery fat that goes easily. I usually notice that men lose weight quicker in the first four weeks than women but women eventually lose more than the men.

If a health issue like a cold should attack you, and after spraying nose and throat frequently with an antiseptic, and denying the cold vigorously, it persists in running it's course, better go back to your maintenance diet for a few days.

Don't "taste"! You will find the second taste much harder to resist than the first. If you have allowed in your daily program something between meals (a good plan), take it, but not otherwise.

Try not to overeat at any time, and thus undo the work that perhaps has taken you two or three days to accomplish. I notice that if I eat slowly and I become full. I sigh or take a large breath. That tells me it's time to stop eating so I just bag or box the rest and have it for lunch or dinner the next day. Remember, It will be all right occasionally, possibly one day a week, to eat up to your maintenance diet, but don't, I beg of you, go over it. If you do you gain the weight and negate the diet completely.

Without hypnotherapy, you will be tempted quite frequently, and you will have to choose whether you will enjoy yourself hugely in the twenty minutes or so that you will be consuming the excess calories, or whether you will dislike yourself cordially for the two or three days you lose by your lack of will power. That is why I highly recommend clinical hypnotherapy. It will curb those urges and will make you full so you do not want that extra food.

9

My Thin Friends Advise

I did not give our thin friends a sample menu for fear it would upset them; but nothing can upset your digestion, I know. However, I will not give you a sample menu, either, but will tell you what I eat when I go on a reduction regime, which for me is 1200 Calories each and every day. I tried less, much less and I needed food. I looked like I was sick. I was however, very weak all of the time.

I have noticed, most of my calories I have at dinner in the evening. It is actually more healthy to have your larger caloric intake during the mid day meal. You may not like this, but would rather have yours spread over the entire day; and you can suit your self, for it makes no difference as long as your total number per day stays within your reduction limit.

Fat seems to melt faster when the chief meal is in the middle of the day, and with only 200 or 300 calories of fruit for the evening meal. In this way you slim while you sleep.

I usually have a bowl of cereal in the morning and if I have a meal at lunch time I'll have my protein motion milkshake at dinner, if I have my protein milkshake at lunch time that I have a meal for dinner. I use self hypnosis on myself in order to eliminate the hunger pangs and not be constantly hungry. I also snack on apples and other fruits when I just need a boost.

Make Out Several Menus if You Like

Don't think you have to follow my menu. You might gain on it! Study the Key and select your own.

Many will lose by going on the no-breakfast plan, or the no-lunch plan. If they do reduce, it is because they have lowered their daily consumption of food, and not because of the no-breakfast or no-lunch plan *per SE. I do not recommend the no breakfast plan for the simple reason that if your body does not have the food or the fat. It will go into starvation mode and save or store the fat. So I tell you that it's hard to lose weight. If your body is storing the fat. , I do not recommend the no breakfast plan. Breakfast is your most important meal.*

MY BREAKFAST

usually, one bowl of many wheat cereal using 2% milk. Occasionally I'll have two pieces of toast with butter, (not margarine), toast, butter and jelly with a glass of 2% milk. This will last me until lunchtime.

You may prefer many more calories for breakfast, or none at all. This may not look good to you, but it means an awful lot to me, after my exercise and shower, to sit down to my little breakfast and read my emails.

Recently I have found that two cups of moderately hot water with the juice of a lemon answers just as well as the toast , and is probably better. You might like some fruit with your breakfast.

MY LUNCH

for lunch it depends on if I'm at home or away from the house. If I'm at home I can select from many items in the fridge. and basically it depends on how hungry I am either have a peanut butter and jelly sandwich 275 cal in a glass of 2% milk 80 cal. Or I'll just have my milkshake. I protein milkshake that I discussed earlier calories. Unknown. I usually try a small salad if I am not having my shake.

If you are constipated, substitute one bran muffin. Since I've been drinking my milk shakes. I have never been constipated. You can see that this is in reality a further extension of my sumptuous breakfast.

You might prefer a baked apple or two tomatoes, or a dish of prunes, or 3 oz. of cottage cheese. The main thing is to take what you like, not what I like. Count your calories.

MY DINNER

well for dinner if I had my milkshake for lunch then I pretty much eat anything I want for dinner. I just eat small amounts and watch my calories. I don't snack in between meals, and I don't snack after dinner.

SUMMARY

Breakfast 75 C.

Lunch including salad 355 C.

 Dinner 700 C. -------

Total for the day , estimated at 1130 C.

That leaves me 50 more calories to total 1200, to take before going to bed . You should leave this 50 calories to take before retiring, because if you are hungry you will find it very difficult to go to sleep. Remember to hydrate throughout the day, with water. I suggest a large glass when you first get out of bed in the morning, a large class approximately half hour before each meal and a large class right before you go to bed at night (unless it will make you get up several times at night) to keep the body hydrated and you sleep more comfortably. And if you like . Instead at night a small cup of warm skimmed milk tends to be a sedative. Hunger, like cold feet, is hard to go to sleep on.

If there is one thing more important than another, it is thorough mastication. Which basically means Chewing your food.

This applies to the thin as well as to the fat, and to the child as well as to the adult. Take a moderate mouthful and work with it until it is automatically swallowed. Chew slowly until it is all gone before you put any more in your mouth. There is no better way of making yourself think that you have had all you want than this habit, and it takes the same time to consume one-half the amount of food you have been in the habit of eating. If you eat slowly, you'll burn more calories and you will realize when you're full and not overeat.

I will allow you all the water you want, in reason; in fact, I advise it while you are reducing, both at the meals and between meals. The only precaution is that at the meals it should not be drunk while food is in the mouth, for this would tend to lessen proper digestion of the food. Remember, drink your water approximately half hour before the meal. Digesting begins in the mouth, not the stomach like most people think.

Now, when are you going to begin this important business of reducing? After the holidays? Tomorrow? *No! Right now.* Get out the phone book look up hypnotherapy call a clinical hypnotherapist and set an appointment do it now because the sooner you get started, the better. The chief thing to do, and the hardest, is to get started and to get the habit. After the first couple of days you will not dread it; in fact; you will feel so much better that you will not be willing to go back to your old habits of overeating.

Now let's review a bit what you are to do.

First: locate and call a clinical hypnotherapist and set an appointment, then pledge to yourself, and to someone else, so you will be ashamed to fail. There is a great deal of psychology to reducing. Use strong auto-suggestion. Decide just how much you are going to eat in advance of the meal--so many calories, *no more!* This sounds foolish, but it helps wonderfully. Set a goal. eg. By Dec. 1st I will weigh x number of pounds.

Second: Begin with a fast or a low caloric diet for the first day; keep it, if necessary, one day weekly.

Third: Study food list and make out menus the caloric totals of which *are less* than your maintenance diet. Have a fairly balanced diet, some fat, some carbohydrates, some protein, and a good amount of green vegetables and fruit. *Have 200-300 C's of protein.*

Fourth: slowly chew every morsel with such thoroughness that it is automatically swallowed. Take twice the amount of time to eat as you normally would.

Fifth: Keep up your activities and other volunteer work, or walk to work bicycled work get off the bus at a different stop and walk further.

Sixth: Remember that you will feel good in your little heart when you resist temptation to overeat, and when you don't, you won't feel good anywhere.

Seventh: Start some type of exercise program. Remember to check with your doctor first if you have health issues.

NOTE: If there comes a time when you think you will die unless you have some chocolate creams, do self hypnosis as instructed by your hypnotherapist. Or make yourself a bowl of clear soup 25 C. 1 cracker 25 C. ------ Total 50 C.

And thus, you see, every supposed pleasure in sin (eating) will furnish more than its equivalent of pain (dieting) until belief in material life (chocolate creams) is destroyed.

Review

1. Describe your stomach.

2. If there is one thing more important than another, what is it?

3. Repeat the five orders in chapter 8.

4. Repeat the warnings.

5. Work the following example:

X gains 25 pounds during the year. How many calories has he averaged daily over his maintenance diet?

KEY:

25 lbs. fat = 400 oz. fat. 1 oz. fat represents 275 C. food consumed. 400 oz. = 400 x 275, or 110,000 C. 110,000 ÷ 365 = 301 C. *Answer.* X has eaten 301 C. per day more than necessary.

6. How many calories have you averaged daily over your maintenance diet? And what could you have left off your menu and kept from gaining all that weight?

10

Testimonials

After you have reduced or gained, let me share your joys. Write me a little note. You need not sign your name if you don't want to. Send an email to walker@wnchypnotherapy.com

11

An Apology and Some Amendments

Some Amendments

You perhaps have noticed that my first chapter is called "Preliminary Bout," I am aware that P.B. is a prize fighting term, and I meant it for the fact that losing weight at the beginning sometimes is a fight, especially without hypnotherapy.

12

Maintenance Diet and Conclusions

A daily diet containing more than necessary for maintenance; for example, let us say 1000 calories more will make you gain weight because you will store fat. This 1000 calories of food is equivalent to approximately 4 ounces of fat [1000÷255 (1 oz. fat = 255 C.)]; 4 ounces of fat daily equals 8 pounds a month which will be added to your weight, and, if not needed by the system and your body will deposit itself as excess fat.

Or the toxins arising from the unnecessary food will irritate the blood vessels, causing arterial-sclerosis (hardening of the arteries), which in turn may cause kidney disease, heart disease, or apoplexy (rupture of artery in the brain), and maybe death before your time.

On the other hand, if you are underweight and the added nourishment is gradually worked up to, it will improve the health and cause a gain of so much (theoretically, and in reality if kept up long enough).

Now the diet containing less than the maintenance; again, for example, say 1000 calories less. Here the 1000 calories must be taken from the body tissue, and fat is the first to go, for fat is virtually dead tissue.

This 4 ounces of fat daily which will be supplied by your body and equals in six months 48 pounds.

There are in America hundreds of thousands of overweight individuals; not all so much overweight as this, but some considerably more so. If these individuals will save 1000 calories of food daily by using their stored fat, think what it would mean at this time.

If, as discussed in previous parts of this book, if 1000 calories or less is eaten and the individual already is underweight, with no excess fat, then this amount will be taken from the muscles and the more vital tissues, and the organism will finally succumb. Before this time is reached there will be a great lowering of resistance, and the individual will be more susceptible to infectious diseases.

It must be remembered that in children the growth of the whole body is tremendously active, and especially that of the heart and nervous system.

If the nervous system is undernourished, it becomes disorganized and undeveloped. This is apt to be expressed in uncertain emotional states, quick tempers, and a predisposition to convulsions. The heart, if undernourished, lays its foundation for future heart disease, and the whole system will be injured for life.

Anything that impairs the vigor and vitality of children strikes at the basis of national welfare.

You can see from this how extremely important it is that, in our need for the conservation of food, only those who can deny themselves and at the same time improve their health and efficiently should do it. It will be no help in our crisis if the health and resistance of our people be lowered and the growth and development of our children be stunted.

13

It is better while you are reducing to stay away from the dining table when you do not expect to eat. If you are living in a small apartment, get a tiny coffee maker, some tea or coffee, some cream substitute, and you can make a hot drink in your apartment and be independent for your breakfast and your evening meal, when you decide some day to go without that. Do not take more than 100 calories for your breakfast. That leaves you 1100 calories to be divided during the day if you go on a 1200 calorie schedule. I suggest the following distribution of the calories:

Breakfast 100 C's.

Lunch 350 " Tea 100 "

Dinner 650 "

You can reverse the dinner and lunch if you desire. If you do so then have your 100 calories I have allowed for tea time to take just before you retire. On a 1200 calorie schedule arranged as I have it you will not be hungry, I assure you. It will not be more than three or four days before your stomach will be shrunk and this amount I have allowed you will almost seem like overeating! That is the big idea. Shrink your stomach. Go on a fast or low calorie day, for a whole day if necessary to get started.

I can safely say that any adult who is up and around will reduce on 1200 calories a day, that amount will not supply the basal metabolism, i.e., the body's internal activities, such as the beating of the heart, respiration, digestion, excretion, etc., and some of the body's stored fat will be called upon to supply the deficiency. How much one will reduce depends on how many calories are actually needed for the internal and the external activities. It is not advisable to lose weight too rapidly. I tell my hypnotherapy clients that a goal of 2 pounds a month is an acceptable goal. Most of you would agree that 2 pounds is a gosl that can be accomplished without trying too hard.

Now you have 1200 calories a day to eat. Let us think of this in terms of money. You have a limited amount of money every day to spend for food. You must spend it judiciously and get the food you need and want. If you spend the most of it on one article you have that much less for other things. It is possible that some days you will want to spend more than your allowance and you draw on your next day's supply. That will be all right if you remember that you have done so and will spend that much less the next day to equalize your account. You must study to spend wisely and carefully so as to supply your needs, but you cannot spend more than you have. The same goes for calories. Remember what you take in on calories is all you have. Calories in calories out.

I wish you great success with your weight loss program and remember the first thing I suggest that you need to do is to contact a clinical hypnotherapist set up an appointment and follow their exact program. I suggest that you find one that is a member of a international association like the National Guild of Hypnosis. I am a proud member and I know that they are a credible organization.

If hypnotherapy is not what you will do then eat a well-balanced diet, and start an exercise program. That's all there is to it. If you're remembering count your calories. Do the age and calorie count so that you know how much you should take in. You should be able to lose weight if you follow the steps above. Remember, If you can change the way you think, you can change your destiny.

The end, or a new beginning. Your Choice.

God bless and happy thinning.

www.ingramcontent.com/pod-product-compliance
Lightning Source LLC
Chambersburg PA
CBHW050754290526
45792CB00008B/2181